TABLE OF CONTENTS

Introduction

Life is filled with choices, our choices affect us and others in dramatic ways whether we see it immediately or not. We have got so busy chasing the new shiny object and getting validation from others. I mean it seems foolish to keeping your focus on **"shiny tiles but not looking at bugs underneath."** Or **"Focus on the party on titanic don't look at the iceberg, the party is on titanic. Look at the titanic."**

Anybody who gets his mind diverted from what is important and valuable is doomed to suffer health problems. We need to change this way of thinking and treat our body as the most important physical equipment in the world, because from your point of view it is. I say this because everything depends on your health, wealth is no good if you neglect your health. You cannot enjoy the riches you gained by sheer hard work, due to poor health problems.

Have you wondered why some people can eat what they want without ever gaining a pound? Well, you are not alone, I also did. The secret lies in the science of thermodynamics and insulin resistance which is covered in this book.

There are many reasons why people are overweight but the great news is that it can all go and fairly quickly too. We live in a world full of information but some of the information is manipulated by corporations with monetary interest who brainwash us into buying their junk they brand as healthy food. You are holding in your hand an opportunity to achieve your dream body without you having to starve, buy expensive supplements or do any crazy fad diets.

This book will cover practical tips and tricks on why and how to get rid of the weight, lose the fat not only for aesthetic reasons but also for health reasons, an example being lowering of blood pressure and reversing the top ten leading causes of death. If your weight is a concern and you want to quickly lose the weight, this book is for you. So this is it, the complete practical guide to what it takes to lose weight and gain your perfect body. The plan to attain all your health and fitness desires is found in the book you are holding, so read on and let it shake your world.

Chapter 1 - Why do you need to eat healthily?

"Treat your body like a temple, not a wood shed"

If I gave you your favourite car (for example Lamborghini) and told you, you are only going to have this one car for the rest of your life. I am 110% sure that you would look after that car and make sure it's running optimally.

Pop Quiz - How many physical bodies do you have in life?
Answer = 1. You are going to have one physical body for life so it makes perfect sense to learn how to look after it and make sure it runs effectively. Health issues can put a massive strain on your overall personal development, success and ability to enjoy your life. Imagine if your friends and family go skiing or go on a roller coaster but you cannot because you are overweight. As the old saying goes treat your body like a temple, not a wood shed.

What are the benefits of a healthy lifestyle?
A healthy lifestyle has many benefits in both the short and long term, however most people are not aware of all the benefits. Below are some of the key benefits of a healthy lifestyle:

- Increased productivity - Just Like a car, your brain needs quality fuel (food) to run efficiently. When it comes to your job, working more efficiently can help you earn more. High achievers are usually first in line for promotions and raises. In 2012, a study published by Population Health Management found that eating an unhealthy diet puts you at a 66% increased risk of productivity loss. Another study in the Journal of Occupational and Environmental Medicine found that an unhealthy diet represented the highest risk for low productivity out of 19 possible risk factors including lack of exercise, chronic pain and financial instability.

- Money savings on health insurance - Health insurance premiums/bills can be a major drain on your bank account, health insurance premiums are partially based on how healthy you are. The healthier you are, the more you save.

- Combat Diseases - Healthy habits aid in the prevention of health conditions such as heart disease, stroke and high blood pressure. If you follow a healthy diet and exercise correctly, you can keep your cholesterol and blood pressure within a safe range. This keeps your blood flowing smoothly and decreases your risk of cardiovascular diseases. Regular physical activity and a clean diet can also prevent or help manage a wide range of health problems such as:

- Metabolic syndrome
- Diabetes
- Depression
- Various Cancers
- Arthritis

- <u>Improves longevity:</u> When you practice healthy habits you boost your chances of a longer life. Recently I read a report by The American Council on Exercise, within this report, an eight-year study was conducted consisting of 13,000 people. This study showed that those who walked just 30 minutes each day significantly reduced their chances of dying prematurely, compared to those who exercised infrequently. Looking forward to spending more time with loved ones is a reason good enough to keep exercising.

Summary

Being healthy has many advantages, as far as I see it there is no downside. The only challenge is getting moving and becoming active. Especially if you are somebody who naturally is not active. I would like to encourage you to schedule a physical exam every year. Get your doctor to check your weight, heartbeat, blood pressure and take a urine and blood sample. This simple appointment can reveal a lot about your health. It is vital to keep track of your body. It's important to follow up with your doctor and listen to health improvement recommendations. Again going back to the car example, most people get their car serviced every year. But they neglect their body. Do not be like most people as your body is one of the most important assets in life. You only have one body so learn to look after it. By picking up this book, you have already started the process of nurturing your body.

Chapter 2 - The need for change

"We can't solve problems by using the same kind of thinking we used when we created them. "Albert Einstein

The typical western diet has many flaws; the primary flaw is that we consume too many calories which contain too few nutrients. In today's world, fast food is affordable, readily available and a convenient way to fill you up when on the run. Although you shouldn't feel guilty for an occasional indulgence, regularly eating fast food can seriously damage your health.

The major issue is that fast food is low in nutritional value in combination with high fat, calorie and sodium content leading to a variety of health problems. There are numerous statistical studies linking consumption of fast food with weight gain, obesity, diabetes, cardiovascular conditions and all-cause mortality. Regularly eating fast food is not only bad but it is also dangerous.

Most common problems that stem from a poor diet are:
- <u>Digestive and Cardiovascular Systems</u> - Many fast foods and drinks are loaded with carbohydrates and sugar. This equates to a lot of calories. Your digestive system breaks carbohydrates

down into glucose (blood sugar) when blood sugar is high your pancreas responds by releasing insulin which is needed to transport sugar to cells throughout your body. As the sugar is absorbed, your blood sugar levels drop. When blood sugar gets low, your pancreas releases another hormone called glucagon.

Glucagon tells the liver to start making use of stored sugars. This is good when everything is working in sync and blood sugar levels stay within a normal range. When you eat high amounts of carbohydrate it causes a spike in your blood sugar which alters the normal insulin response. Frequent spikes in blood sugar are a major factor in type 2 diabetes risk.

- <u>Sugar</u> - Added sugars have no nutritional value but are high in calories. According to the American Heart Association most Americans consume twice the recommended servings for sugar. All those extra calories add up and cause you to put on extra weight which is a major factor for heart disease risk.
- <u>Fat</u> – Trans-fats are a manufactured fat with no extra nutritional value. Trans-fats are considered so unhealthy that some countries have banned their use. However, still we see people day in day out queuing at fast food chains. Trans-fats are also known to raise LDL cholesterol levels. LDL cholesterol is the undesirable kind of cholesterol and can also lower HDL

cholesterol which is the good cholesterol. Trans-fats may also increase your risk of developing type 2 diabetes.

- <u>Sodium</u> - Sodium is a key reason why so many people feel bloated and puffy after eating at a restaurant. Restaurants tend to add high amounts of sodium and sugar into their meals as high amounts of sodium and sugar are very addictive to humans. Too much sodium causes your body to retain water hence making you feel bloated, puffy and appear fatter. But that's the least of the damage that overly salted foods can do to our body. If you have congestive heart failure, cirrhosis or kidney disease too much salt can contribute to a dangerous build-up of water retention. Excess sodium can increase your risk for kidney stones, kidney disease and stomach cancer. According to research high cholesterol and high blood pressure are among the top risk factors for heart disease and stroke.

In 2015 a report commissioned by "Beat" estimates more than 725,000 people in the UK are affected by an eating disorder. Eating disorders tend to be more common in certain age groups but they can affect people of any age. Eating disorders include a range of conditions that can affect someone physically, psychologically and socially. The most common types of eating disorders are:

- <u>Anorexia nervosa</u> – A psychological disorder characterized by an obsession to keep weight as low as possible by starvation or excessive exercise. In a 2015 report commissioned by Beat around 1 in 250 women and 1 in 2,000 men will experience anorexia nervosa at some point in their lives. This is more common in young women however with new diet fads many other/new individuals are joining this unhealthy bandwagon.

- Bulimia – When a person goes through periods of binge eating to get deliberately sick or uses laxatives (medication to help empty the bowels) to try to control their weight by throwing up all the food ingested. This condition most commonly develops around the age of 16 or 17. Bulimia is around two to three times more common than anorexia nervosa and 90% of people with this condition are female.

- Binge eating disorder (BED) – When a person feels compelled to overeat large amounts of food in a short space of time. Binge eating equally affects males and females and usually appears later in life, between the ages of 30 and 40. It's difficult to precisely define binge eating, it's not clear how widespread it is. But it's estimated to affect around 5% of the adult population.

What causes eating disorders?

Eating disorders are often blamed on the social pressure to be thin. Most young people are socially conditioned via TV, parents and environment to look a particular way. If an individual does not look the way they are expected to look, the individual feels stress, discomfort and isolation, this causes negative emotions leading to depression.

An eating disorder can be associated with biological, genetic or environmental factors combined with a particular event that triggers the disorder. There can also be other factors which cause an Individual to keep suffering from the disorder. Factors increasing the likelihood of eating disorders include:

- Having a family history of eating disorders, depression or substance misuse.
- Being criticised for their eating habits, body shape or weight.
- Being overly concerned with being slim, particularly if combined with pressure to be slim from society or for a job – for example, ballet dancers, models or athletes.
- Underlying characteristics, examples include: having an obsessive personality, an anxiety disorder, low self-esteem or being a perfectionist.
- Life experiences, such as sexual or emotional abuse or the death of someone special.
- Difficult relationships with family members or friends.
- Stressful situations – for example, problems at work, school or university.

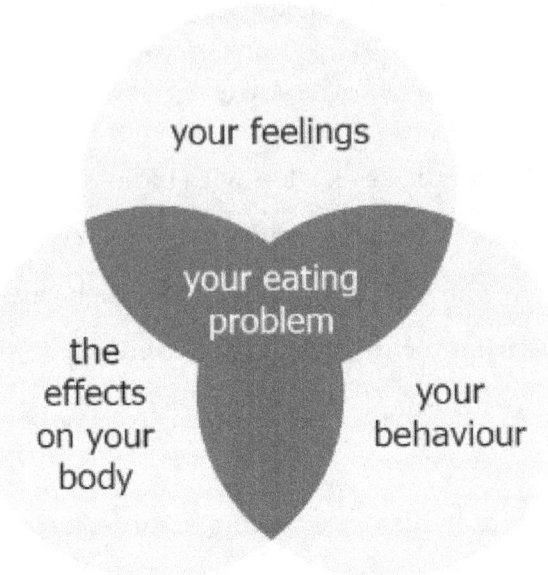

Summary

Now that you understand the flaw in our current way of eating and the impact it can have on our life. Our eating habits are at the core of our behaviour as well as the condition of our body. I hope this chapter showed you the flaw and helped you understand why we need to change our diet. If you want more motivation, just picture yourself, eating fast food for the whole year or even 2 years.

- How would you look?
- How would you feel in your body?
- How would it affect your brain or productivity rating?
- How would your partner feel about being with you?
- Do you think you will be setting a good example for your kids or Family members?

Chapter 3 – The science of gaining fat

This chapter explains why we get fat as well as discussing the challenges of mainstream thinking, which blames obesity on eating too much and moving too little. Different foods have different hormonal and metabolic responses on the human body. We have always been told that obesity is a person's fault for eating too much and moving too little but this is not necessarily the truth.

Fact: Insulin resistance

Different foods produce different metabolic and hormonal responses for example carbohydrates produce more of the hormone insulin in comparison to any other macronutrient. Insulin is the fat storage hormone and acts as a gatekeeper to fat storage. Carbohydrates are quickly converted to glucose i.e. blood sugar, once blood sugar is spiked the excess energy cannot be handled by the human body and therefore must be stored as fat. This is where insulin comes into play, insulin the hormone is used to push the excess blood sugar into our fat cells, making us fat!

There are 3 storage forms that carbohydrates converted to glucose can take up within the body when sugar is spiked.

- The first is within the liver, the liver stores a limited amount of energy and your liver "tank" is rather small.

- The second storage area is glucose which can fill up is our muscles. Muscle fibre can store more glucose in comparison to the liver but still a finite amount that can easily be spiked if a steady supply of glucose is not received.
- The third storage form that glucose energy can take is within fat cells, when excess energy cannot be stored within muscles they must be stored as fat.

Greater insulin production means more fat will be stored, with time our bodies becoming increasingly resistant to insulin's message to the body which causes more insulin (fat storage hormone) to be produced as our body isn't responding to insulin's message and therefore needs to produce more of it. This vicious downward spiral often leads to health problems. Remember this only occurs when blood sugar is spiked. Different foods raise blood sugar (glucose) at different rates.

The macronutrient fat only very slightly raises blood sugar; proteins only slightly raise blood sugar. Whereas refined carbs and sugars send blood sugar skyrocketing, therefore producing more fat storage hormone making us fat. Insulin and high blood sugar (glucose) are also what contributes to mid-afternoon tiredness or causes post-meal tiredness. So carbohydrates produce the most insulin but we do need some carbohydrate in our diet for our day-to-day functionality and for energy reasons. Therefore, it is important to correctly balance blood sugar levels.

Calories in vs out

Not all calories are created equally. To prove this concept, I give you two different example meals:

30 teaspoons of pure refined sugar (500 calories) vs 37oz broccoli (500 calories)

Which meal will lead to greater weight gain?

Well. There will be a huge difference in how your body absorbs pure refined sugar in comparison to how broccoli is stored and processed within the body. Apart from being completely unhealthy, the calories from sugar will cause more weight gain due to more of the fat storage hormone insulin being produced. Calorie count does matter but keep into consideration that you have "good" calories and "bad" calories.

Summary

Now that you have a better understanding of how different foods produce different metabolic and hormonal responses. Carbohydrates produce more of the hormone insulin, Insulin is the fat storage hormone and acts as a gatekeeper to fat storage.

Not all calories are created equally, there are good quality calories and bad calories. Just because you consumed the recommended amount doesn't mean you will stay lean and healthy, you have to consume good quality calories. I can consume 2000 calories from McDonald's and get my recommended dose but those calories are not good in quality & nutrients.

Chapter 4 – FULL Responsibility + NO Excuses = 100% RESULTS

For a fair share of my life, at least 20 years I *"CHOSE"* to be 30 pounds' overweight. Now the reason why I say I *"CHOSE"* to be, it is because I never accidently ate that Big Mac or KFC Big Daddy meal. It was always a choice. I mean I could have said no, but all the time I gave into short term gratification and rationalised my decision.

So as you go on reading this book, if you are overweight I want you to take *FULL RESPONSIBILITY* for being overweight. Stop pointing the finger at your family, friends, society, work, peers or big foot. The way you look and feel in life, it is 100% due to your decisions, choices and actions. The sooner you accept this fact the quicker you can change or fix the situation or circumstances you are in.

"Accountability breeds responsibility.

Stephen Covey"

Prevention is better than cure - WHY?

Prevention is better than a cure because it literally prevents the discomfort and costs of becoming sick or experiencing a similar preventable event. It also often takes less effort to prevent something than to cure it hence the popular expression **"an ounce of prevention is worth a pound of cure"** this originally came from Benjamin Franklin.

Common prevention strategies such as regular hand washing help prevent illnesses like cold and flu from spreading. If you simply take some time to plan & prepare your food you can prevent food poisoning from fast food and excessive weight gains due to the food being high in sugar, salt and fats.

In both cases, it is much more efficient and cost-effective to prevent the problem than to cure it. Taking the time to prevent a negative scenario from happening, whether it is gaining fat or experiencing a careless accident. Prevention is always better than dealing with the scenario after it occurs. Eating healthy isn't always easy, but committing to a healthy eating plan can be one of the smartest decisions you EVER make.

Why?

Not only can eating well make you look and feel better, it can also save you money on future health costs. I want you to remember the simple formula below as you are presented with a chance to consume fast food.

Garbage in = Garbage out

Quality food in = Quality work out

Summary

This was a short chapter on renewing your perspective. The key takeaway from this chapter is that your health is your responsibility and only yours, not your moms, dads or friends. The quicker you pick up the responsibility the quicker you can get the results you want.

The second major takeaway is: Prevention is better than cure. It is much better to prevent yourself from gaining 30 pounds then it is trying to lose it. If you are overweight, please don't worry because later in the book I will help you put together a plan of action which you can follow to lose weight and get your desired body. But I want you to make a commitment and promise to yourself that from this day forward:

"You are in control of your health and take 100% responsibilities for how you look physically"

Chapter 5 - MYTH vs FACT = Always work with FACTS

You will find tons of ridiculous health claims on the internet and some are actually believable. These days it seems like everything makes you fat apart from gluten-free food which is the key to eternal youth but you will need to poop ten times a day or you will die. I am obviously joking, but today we are going to look at some of the common myths and uncover the truth.

MYTHS vs FACT #1- Eat six small meals a day for fat loss

This theory is based on the calories in vs calories out myth. If we divide 2000 calories by 6. It's a (2000/6) mere 330 calories per meal. This is very limiting in itself as, you are never satisfied with the amount eaten and therefore you never feel full. Anybody who believes this myth is more likely to over eat the extra amount during the snacking.

For the person doing Intermittent Fasting i.e. only eating twice a day. It is extremely difficult to consume 2000 calories in the space of two meals, especially with protein as your body will give you a fullness signal before the 1000+ calories are consumed.

Again this comes back to what is natural, I don't think Caveman would ration out six equal protein meals to eat at specifically balanced times. The greater likelihood is that Caveman would spend all day hunting for food and then bring back rewards of the day's hunt back to the tribe or colony.

Frequent eating and breakfast are now only modern revolutions, fasting has been practiced widely by many major world religions. But why do I feel so drained when I skip breakfast? Well, as your body has adjusted to eating every 2-3 hours it expects and receives food, therefore once you refrain from breakfast your body adapts by producing less Ghrelin which is the hormone your body uses to tell you that it is hungry. Overall intermittent fasting is a great fat loss tool. Don't believe me? Try it for yourself.

MYTH vs FACT #2 - Under eating causes you to hold onto fat

If you under eat you will lose fat, if you constantly under eat every day you will still lose fat.

There is a popular myth that if you under eat your body will hold onto fat, case and point the Minnesota Starvation Experiment. This was an experiment where participants we're literally starved whilst they over-exercised and under ate. Respondents stopped losing fat after a certain period however they only stopped losing fat when their fat levels reached dangerously low levels. So yes your body will hang on to fat only if there is very little of it.

So why should you not under eat if this is the case? The answer is simply health and muscle loss. Participants in the starvation experiment also lost muscle, became very dizzy and disturbingly ill. It's simply not a healthy way to lose weight.

What is also not clear is how the participants would respond to weight regain, an example of this is reality TV series shows such as "Extreme Weight Loss" where contestants spend hours on end exercising and also eating very little for months on end. They always lose weight. But do they do it in a healthy way? Maybe.

There was a case of a man named 'Rod Durham' who was a contestant on "Extreme Weight Loss", the high school English teacher lost 180 lbs on the ABC show. Just two years after losing the weight Rod Durham died as a result of diabetic shock which was linked to his rapid weight loss, Rod Durham's tragic story isn't the only case. Therefore, it is quite important to seek professional advice when taking anything to the extreme.

MYTH or FACT - Gaining Muscle for Men and Women

Body composition affects fat, the more muscle you equip the lower your relative body fat is making you appear leaner as your body fat to muscle ratio is decreased. Muscle building is a very difficult and slow process; men typically don't mind the extra muscle but women fear muscle may make them appear bulky. As for women, I assure you it will not make you look bulky at all. This is because women cannot naturally put on a huge amount of muscle and if anything added muscle makes women look more toned and curvy.

Gaining muscle will also make you feel better, burn more calories at rest and make you a lot stronger overall, with more muscle you will also be able to defend yourself much better in the event of conflict. There are many benefits to increasing muscle mass and it is important for men and even for women. Strength training will literally change your life as it will help in your day to day functionality, athleticism, attraction, confidence and self-belief. I cannot stress this enough. So make sure you lift weights, rest and eat enough protein.

MYTH or FACT - Sleep for Fat Loss

The science is unclear on whether broken sleep itself makes you gain or lose weight. What is clear is when your body is sleep deprived your much more likely to skip exercise and workouts, due to being more tired or not cooking clean, healthy meal and ordering a takeout instead. This links back to energy, sleep is very important for health and your fat loss motivation efforts. Be sure to sleep in a cold, dark, quiet room and to avoid any bright lights hours before bed. Let your body wind down with a hot bath before bedtime, remember better sleep will correlate in greater fat loss.

Summary

We live in world full of information however, the validity of the information is difficult to confirm. Especially with the power of the internet there are always countless new diets fads being released. But it's only when you start questioning what you are being told and start seeing the world through your eyes, you start seeing what is valid and what is bullshit. As humans, we learn 2 ways:

- <u>First-hand Experience</u> – When you do something yourself and learn. For example, I burned my finger while cooking so I have first-hand experience and learned to not touch hot things as I know they can burn my hand.
- <u>Second-hand Experience</u> – When somebody else has done something and you can learn from their experience. For example, I know if I jump out the window from the 20th floor, chances are I will die. I do not have any first-hand experience but I know from second-hand experience that this is sound knowledge.

There are pros and cons to both sides of the coin of 1st hand and 2nd experience. The second-hand information is extremely helpful as it saves us time and energy. However, the problem is when you start taking bad/failed second-hand information from society, our parents or the internet.

I believe we must learn to see the world through our own eyes. Take the second-hand information, ponder it, analyse it and make sure the conclusion you reach is based on your judgement and your judgement alone. For example, if my negative uncle tells me exercising is a waste of time because you won't see any change. My uncle says this because he has trained and dieted for over a year but he doesn't see any results. I can believe this second-hand information but if I question it. Is there anyone in history who has dieted and exercised and saw positive results?

The answer is yes. Because I have questioned the information and now I can make a better judgement. I want to encourage you to question every second-hand information that comes into your life regarding diet or exercise. The second experience is good as it saves time and energy. But question the second-hand information as much as you can before buying into the information.

When I turned 19, I wanted to become a bouncer but everybody told me I can't do it. Everybody gave me countless reasons, that I was too small, not strong enough, not fast enough, not smart, you will get beaten up etc. But I refused to listen and applied for a 'Security Industry Association license'. Once I got my license, I worked in different pubs, clubs, and festivals. I got to see some of my favourite celebrities such as Drake, Bruno Mars, and Tom Jones. I loved every bit of working in the security industry but if I didn't get the first-hand experience I would have believed that I can't do it.

First-hand experience is the quickest way to learn skills and cut down the learning curve. A great example is if you want to learn how to swim the best way to learn is to dive into the pool and try swimming. You can sit on the internet and watch different videos about techniques and read different articles. The same principal applies to your health, just starting taking action and educating yourself about the field. The positive results will follow.

To summarize it is not one size fits all for weight loss, some people benefit from eating smaller more frequent meals and some people benefit from intermittent fasting, my advice to you is to experiment. The best way to learn is to take massive action and dive straight into the pool, rather than tip-toeing into the pool. Life is too short to do that.

Chapter 6 - Renovation

Are you on a diet at the moment?

Well good for you, so are millions of other women and men all around the world. But the statistics show that the vast majority (a staggering 95 percent) won't manage to lose weight and keep it off.

So why do 95% of diets fail?

Now there are a countless reason's why diets fail. But after in-depth research, below are the KEY reasons why MOST diets fail.

PROBLEM # Your diet is too strict - Lack of flexibility

Most people get a professional trainer or nutritionist to make them a diet plan however, the issue is most of the time their diet is too strict. The diet bans all your favourite foods (chocolate, cheese, ice cream, chips) and you feel deprived. You might last a couple of weeks, feeling more and more bored with the tedious repetition of your regime but sooner or later, you will crack. And when you do give in, you end up stuffing yourself with those forbidden foods to make up for days of self-denial. Before you know it you are back to square one where you started.

SOLUTION # Balance

Strive for balance in your diet. Hell, I want you to delete the word diet from your vocabulary and call it an "EATING PLAN". If you are new to healthy eating do not set yourself up for failure by copying the Arnold Schwarzenegger, Beyoncé or Kim Kardashian diet routine. The trouble with following the diet of another person is that it is not one size fits all. The person you are following may have the physical body which you aspire to have but they have different genetics and biology to you.

Have you ever worn a tailored made suit?
If you have, you will know it is different from buying the set size from a shopping mall. The way you walk, talk and sit or stand in your tailored suit is different. It is the same with your eating plan. I would say to overcome the problem of strict diet, give yourself some flexibility or balance. A small chocolate bar or a single bag of chips won't ruin your diet. Just like eating one apple or one workout will not make you healthy. Allow yourself to have an occasional treat especially at the start of the eating plan. Once you have followed the plan for 30 to 60 days you can be bit stricter. Once you have tailor made an eating plan you will more likely to stick to it and see results as it is designed for you. It is designed with your goal in mind and it is based on your biology.

PROBLEM #You see your diet as a temporary fix
This is perhaps one of the most frustrating things I see in the gym day in day out. I meet people who successfully managed to lose weight in the past for a special occasion or event. But they inevitably return to

their old eating habits straight afterwards and pile the weight back on. The reason for this issue is that people see dieting or eating healthy as a quick fix rather than a permanent change to make their lifestyle healthier.

SOLUTION #Master the art of consistently

"It's not what we do once in a while that shapes our lives. It's what we do consistently."

Anthony Robbins

For anything to be effective in life, you must do it consistently whether it is working out, eating healthy or playing an instrument etc. Almost all activities in life require consistency in order to bring about change. You must repeat the activity consistently in order to see change. If you take a look at athletes, most people are rendered speechless by their talents and appearances, for example, Ronaldo, Usain Bolt or Tiger Woods. But what most people don't see is the day in day out training. Athletes have mastered the art of being consistent. This is more of a difference in mindset, the people who see dieting as a quick fix have more of an instant gratification mindset. These type of people always look for a quick fix, pill, secret or shortcut.

I am sure we all know someone who has tried the latest diet fad before going on holidays in an attempt to lose some weight quick, there are gazillions of fads on the internet. After applying the fad, the person managed to lose 15 pounds but soon as they returned from their holidays they gain back the 15 pounds along with 10 pounds more. This is one of the universal rules because every goal has process. Whatever you want in life, it has some kind of process. For e.g.

- If you want to become a doctor the process is you go to medical school for x amount of years.
- If you want to become a Lawyer, you go study at law school and practise at a law firm.

Do not try to cheat the system by not following the process because it will come and bite you in the ass. Today's world we have become extremely impatient and want everything quick. Everybody looks for a shortcut or quicker process to acquire the same results as someone who followed the process for years. I had a few friends, whom rather than work out 4-5 days for a couple of months to put on some lean muscle, they simply decided the cut the whole process short by using steroids. This may help you get quicker results but at what cost. If you abuse steroids, you can:

- Develop breasts
- Get painful erections
- Have their testicles shrink
- Have decreased sperm count
- Become infertile
- Become impotent

My advice is not to find shortcuts. As the old saying goes:

"The best things in life are often difficult to come by. It's worth the wait."

I would like to encourage you to use your eating plan as a great excuse to go out and explore different types of foods, change your tastes and find ways of eating healthily that you want to stick to for good. I used to always eat Indian food but now I try a variety of cuisines. This makes eating healthy fun for me. We live in the information age and by using the resources at your fingertips (internet) you can find countless ways to eat healthy and prepare delicious healthy meals. This is all accessible at your fingertips. So if you are serious about losing weight and you are committed and have taken full responsibility of your physical body, you have NO EXCUSE.

PROBLEM #You are too impatient for results from your diet

Once you have made the decision to lose weight, you want it over and done with as soon as possible. When you find that you are losing weight at a rate of one to two pounds a week, you are frustrated: What about all those stories of women shedding 30 pounds in a month? After a couple of weeks, you give up, convinced you are failing because you are not losing weight as fast as you would like to.

SOLUTION # Slow and steady wins the race

Remind yourself that it took months or years to gain that weight. So how can you expect to lose it in weeks or a month time? Remember people who lose weight using fad diets are not likely to keep it off long-term.

If you work slowly but constantly, you will succeed better than if you work fast for a short while and do not continue or worst yet continue after a few months, which is what most people do. You may have seen people at work or gym, who always try the latest diet fad. Which may look like it works but in reality the individual remains the same or at worst gains a little more weight in the end. This is just a vicious downward spiral which often ends with health issues. So whenever you are upset about your results and feel like quitting, remember:

"Slow and steady wins the race"

PROBLEM #Emotions

I believe we as humans are practically programmed from birth to use food emotionally. We bond and celebrate over meals, use food to show our affection, bring others food in times of crisis and use food as a means of comfort. A terrible day at work or a long-awaited promotion may both trigger you to eat. In all the years of my life, I'm certain that overcoming emotional eating is the greatest weight loss hurdle.

SOLUTION # Express yourself

Strong emotions tend to drown out rational thoughts and distance us from the consequences of immediate actions. In simple words, when you are really sad, angry or scared and you know that eating ice cream is going to make you feel better right now.

That's all that matters in the short span of time. It's super easy to push away thoughts about how you will feel tomorrow or detach from goals that aren't relevant in the present moment.

What if I told you, you can change that pattern?

It's not easy, and it doesn't happen overnight, but you can change that pattern. Even if you did not eat emotionally 50, 60 or 70 percent of the time, this shift can have a dramatic impact on your weight. Below are 4 ways that you can use to prevent eating emotionally.

1. **Express yourself**

A friend once told me that her therapist advised her to go to a garage sale or thrift store, buy some cheap dishes, take them into her back yard and smash them to bits. So I asked if she did it?

She said she had, just with one dish and it was one of the most liberating moments of her life. Whether you are walking around with anger, sadness or anxiety bottled up inside, allowing it to fester increases the chances that you will use food to detach or stuff it back down. So for this reason I advise you to find healthy ways to release your feelings, like watching a tearjerker have a good cry or furiously scrubbing the tub to let out aggression. I have used this method it is extremely helpful and efficient. Guaranteed you may seem a little crazy to people who are not aware of what you are doing. But don't worry about them.

"Unexpressed emotions will never die. They are buried alive and will come forth in uglier ways." Sigmund Freud

2. Distance yourself

Over the past few months I've had numerous friends tell me that they can't keep certain foods around, because if they're there, they'll eat them, especially when they're emotional. But unless you live alone, it can be impossible to completely banish all "high risk" foods. One thing that may help is making them harder to get to. Research shows (and my own experience confirms) that the fewer steps you have to go through to get to a food, the more likely you are to eat it and vice versa.

3. Prevent the spiral

One of the biggest challenges many people face is not letting a small indulgence snowball into a big binge. Countless friends who are into eating healthy have told me, "After I went off track, I figured what the heck, I might as well keep eating."

This all or nothing tendency is especially common among people with a history of dieting and ending it. Preventing this can be incredibly transformative, both emotionally and physically. If you are a perfectionistic, it can feel like there's little difference between one "bad" meal and one "bad" day but that's not the truth.

An analogy I use often is debt. If you were on a strict budget to get out of debt, and you spontaneously spent an extra £100, it wouldn't make sense to then go on a spending spree and charge hundreds more to your credit card, right?

If you did, you would just dig a deeper hole that would take longer to get out of, and that's exactly what happens with food. This very pattern is why many people remain roughly the same weight for years, despite constantly being on diets. If that sounds familiar, know that you can break the cycle.

4. Structure your time

For most individuals, the risk of eating emotionally is greater on the weekends, when they have hours of unstructured time. If you are in the same boat, plan a project or activity you enjoy and build in a deadline. For example, if you are making something (jewellery, crafts, etc.), plan to give it to a friend or family member on a specific date. And once you've finished a project, start another. This lifestyle change can result in finally ending what some of my friends refer to as "two-day food orgies" and add to your quality of life in numerous ways.

PROBLEM #Social pressure

Numerous people experience some resistance when they turn down food or drinks because they are trying to eat healthier, friends and family members respond with comments like, "You don't need to lose weight, you look fine." I still get my friends giving me stick for eating salad at restaurants or pulling out my snack pot with almonds and walnuts. One recent study found that friends who eat together consume more food than those paired with strangers. This is because friends give each other "permission" to overeat.

Me and my friends would pig out together on the weekends and have "two-day food orgies". We had to stop as my one of my close buddies suffered a heart attack and was hospitalized. This was wake up call for me and one of the many reasons why I decided to write this book, to create more awareness about the risk of fast food and benefits of a healthy lifestyle.

SOLUTION #Share your goal

Break the eating-as-entertainment pattern. So rather than scheduling social time around a happy hour and dinners out, mix things up. Go to a play rather than a movie, or go out dancing and volunteer to be the designated driver so you can sip on H2O all evening. If you get resistance, concretely explain why your goals are important to you for e.g. eating better helps you sleep, so you are more productive at work, makes your heartburn go away, keeps your migraines at bay…, and ask for friends to support you. Your friends may feel like they have lost a partner in crime, but if they care about you, they'll make peace with adjusting the way you spend time together.

Summary

This chapter was designed to renovate your perspective on diet and some of the most common problems people face. Always remember every problem has a solution, all you have to do it seek the solution.

"Seek and you shall find"

The starting point is always hard; it does not matter what field or industry you are venturing into it. So you must slowly replace all the bad negative thoughts or connatations around diet and train your mind to associate positive thoughts with your health. You will slowly need to dilute your old habits with the new ones.

Image your bad and good habits like the 2 glasses, one full of clean water and one full of dirty water. If you try to dilute the bad habits all at once with good habits, you are doomed to fail. The change will be extremely overwhelming. Just like if I pour the glass of good habits into the bad it will cause the glass to overflow and spill.

You need to need to slowly dilute your current un-serving habits with new ones.

Chapter 7 – Invest in your physical body

"If exercise were a pill, it would be one of the most cost-effective drugs ever invented," Dr. Nick Cavill

Exercise is the miracle cure we have always had it but for too long we have neglected to take our recommended dose. Our health is now suffering as a consequence.

This is no snake oil. Whatever your age, there's strong scientific evidence that being physically active can help you lead a healthier and even happier life.

Health benefits

It seems obvious that we should all be physically active. It's essential if you want to live a healthy and fulfilling life into old age. There are many benefits of regular exercise and maintaining fitness, these include:

- <u>Exercise increases energy levels</u> - Exercise improves both the strength and the efficiency of your cardiovascular system to get the oxygen and nutrients to your muscles. When your cardiovascular system works better everything seems easier and you have more energy for the fun stuff in life.

- <u>Exercise improves muscle strength</u>- Staying active keeps muscles strong and keeps joints, tendons and ligaments flexible. This allows you to move more easily and avoid injury. Strong muscles and ligaments reduce your risk of joint and lower back pain by keeping joints in proper alignment. They also improve coordination and balance.

- <u>Exercise can help you to maintain a healthy weight</u> - The more you exercise, the more calories you burn. In addition, the more muscle you develop, the higher your metabolic rate becomes, so you burn more calories even when you are not exercising. The result? You may lose weight and look better physically which will boost your self-esteem.

- <u>Exercise improves brain function</u> - Exercise increases blood flow and oxygen levels in the brain. It also encourages the release of the brain chemicals (hormones) that are responsible for the production of cells in the hippocampus, the part of the brain that controls memory and learning. This in turn, boosts concentration levels and cognitive ability and also helps reduce the risk of cognitive degenerative diseases such as Alzheimer's.

- <u>Exercise is good for your heart</u> - Exercise reduces LDL cholesterol (the type that clogs your arteries), increases HDL (the good cholesterol) and reduces blood pressure so it lowers the stress on your heart. Adding to this, it also strengthens your heart muscle. Combined with a healthy diet, exercise lowers the risk of developing coronary heart disease. Regular exercise lowers your risk of developing type 2 diabetes. Regular exercise helps to control blood glucose levels, which helps to prevent or delay the onset of type 2 diabetes. Additionally, exercise helps to prevent obesity which is a primary factor in the development of type 2 diabetes.

- <u>Exercise enhances your immune system</u> - Exercise improves your body's ability to pump oxygen and nutrients around your body that are required to fuel the cells that fight bacteria and viruses. Staying active reduces the likelihood of developing some degenerative bone diseases. Weight bearing exercise such as running, walking or weight training lowers your risk of both osteoarthritis and osteoporosis – the adage of **"use it or lose it"** really does apply to bones.

- <u>Exercise may help to reduce the risk of certain cancers</u> - Being fit may mean that the risks of colon cancer, breast cancer and possibly also lung and endometrial cancers are reduced. Studies by the Seattle Cancer Research Centre have suggested that 35% of all cancer deaths are linked to individuals being overweight and inactive. Exercise not only makes you physically fitter but it also improves your mental health and a general sense of well-being.

- <u>Active people tend to sleep better</u> - Physical activity makes you more tired so you are more ready to sleep. Good quality sleep helps improve overall wellness and can reduce stress. Exercise improves your mood and gives you an improved sense of well-being. Physical activity stimulates the release of endorphins which make you feel better and more relaxed. These, in turn, improve your mood and lowers your stress levels.

- <u>Exercise can help prevent and treat mental illnesses like depression</u> - Physical activity can help you meet people, reduce stress levels, cope with frustration, give you a sense of achievement and provide some important **"me time"**, all of which help with depression. Keeping fit can reduce some of the effects of aging.

Summary

Exercising really is the fountain of youth that we are all ought to be drinking from to maintain our health. Based on my perspective it is a no brainer, we should all be exercising. It is an investment which has no downside and great upside.

If we go back to what I said at the start of the book, we as humans are only given one physical body on the earth. Now if you recall I compared the human body to a car and said you only going to have this one car aka one body for life. I am certain if you had one car for life, you would invest time, energy, labour and mental power to ensure that your cars parts are in good health and work efficiently for what you require the car to do?

The same principal applies to your human body is well. You only have one body. I highly recommended that you learn how to fine tune it. When our car breaks down, our first response is to go get the best mechanic and get it fixed.

But with our physical body, we do the freaking opposite. Instead of going to see the doctor or starting an exercise plan, we decided to take chemicals or pharmaceutical pills to mask the problem. This is an extremely dangerous way to treat your body as all you do is mask the problem and suppress it more.

I am sure that we all have met some imbecile, who always brags about his car. You know, **"0 -60 in 3.6666 sec, 500 Horsepower."** Some people value their car so much, spending countless pounds on getting it serviced and adding a new upgrade, new gadgets. But when it comes to looking after their physical health, the person usually looks like pear shaped potato. I am not judging the person based on their appearance, but merely asking a question which is:

- What about your health?
- When was the last you worked out?
- When was the last time you had a medical check-up or invested some money in improving your health?

We have got so busy chasing the new shiny object and getting validation from others. I mean it seems foolish to keeping your focus on **"shiny tiles but not looking at bugs underneath."** Or **"Focus on the party on titanic don't look at the iceberg, the party is on titanic. Look at the titanic."**

Anybody who gets his mind diverted from what is important and valuable is doomed to suffer health problems. We need to change this way of thinking and treat our body as the most important physical equipment in the world, because from your point of view it is. I say this because everything depends on your health, wealth is no good if you neglect your health. You cannot enjoy the riches you gained by sheer hard work, due to poor health problems so by making your body or health a priority, you ensure you achieve your maximum potential in life and have fulfilled life. You will not miss out on any endeavour, adventure or ride, due to the faulty physical body.

Chapter 8 – Exercise HOW WHAT WHY WHERE WHEN?

A modern problem

People are less active nowadays, partly because technology has made our lives easier. We drive cars or take public transport. Machines wash our clothes. We entertain ourselves in front of a TV or computer screen. Fewer people are doing manual work and most of us have jobs that involve little physical effort. Work, house chores, shopping and other necessary activities are far less demanding than for previous generations.

We move around less and burn off less energy than people used to. Research suggests that many adults spend more than seven hours a day sitting down, at work, on transport or in their leisure time. I am IT Engineer and my job involves little to no physical labour. Just like most people I work 40 hours a week, so 40 hours a week I am physically not active so I manage my time and priorities very well. This helps me ensure that I get the recommend minutes of exercise, the week in and week out. People aged over 65 spend 10 hours or more each day sitting or lying down, making them the most sedentary age group.

What counts?

To stay healthy, you should try to be active daily. Your aim should be to achieve at least 150 minutes of physical activity over a week through a variety of activities. This is the bare minimum recommended.

For most people, the easiest way to get moving is to meet the minimum recommended physical exercise. To accomplish this, I encourage you to make an activity a part of everyday life. An activity could be simple as walking or cycling instead of using a car to get around. For any type of activity to benefit your health, you need to be moving quick enough to raise your heart rate, breathe faster and feel warmer. This level of effort is called moderate intensity activity. One way to tell if you are working at a moderate intensity is if you can still talk but you can't sing the words to a song.

If your activity requires you to work even harder, it is called vigorous intensity activity. There is substantial evidence that vigorous activity can bring health benefits over and above that of moderate activity. You can tell when it's vigorous activity because you are breathing hard and fast, your heart rate goes up quite a bit. If you are working at this level, you won't be able to say more than a few words without pausing for a breath.

Types of Activities / Exercises

Different people have different preferences in life and when it comes to exercise this is very applicable. There are different ways to categorize all the different types of activities, I am going to keep my categorization very simple and small. I recommend that you engage in 3 types of exercise/activities. Below are various activities you can engage in:

Stretching

Many people forget to stretch or make the excuse that they don't have the time. Flexibility is important, so make the time! Stretching can be done every day, but stick to a minimum of three times per week in order to reap the benefits. When the body is warmed up, such as after a workout session perform five to ten stretches that target the major muscle groups. Hold each stretch for 10-30 seconds.

Cardio

If you are a beginner, start off slower than you think you should. Three days per week is realistic, safe and effective. If you are experienced, do cardiovascular (aerobic) exercises such as:

- Walking
- Jogging
- Bicycling minimum of 3 hours per week.

<u>Walking</u> - This may seem obvious, but some people may incorporate jogging and sprinting but completely disregard walking as an excellent fat loss tool. The main reason for this is that it can be done every day as a habit, hour on end. Running or Sprinting can become very tiring. You are also always more likely to go for a walk as it's the much easier task in comparison. Walking does not expend as much energy as running, but if you do it more often (which is likely) walking is great. Running and Sprinting are also excellent but this can be very strenuous on overweight people. Other than that there are various health benefits to walking, walking is a great way to get some fresh air and boost your mood, it boosts blood circulation making you more active and it also strengthens your heart.

<u>Pokémon Revolution</u> - You may or may not be aware of the 'Pokémon Revolution', it is a mobile game application where you walk to catch virtual Pokémon. As I write this book, I see a lot of colleagues and friends spending hours and hours of their time, walking and collecting Pokémon. I have not downloaded or tried the game. This is could be low hanging fruit you could use to initiate a commitment to exercise.

Lifting Weights

The minimum recommendation for weight training is no less than three times per week. In this chapter we are going to list some of the most effective exercises to gain strength and build lean muscle. Most of these exercises are compound exercises which you should do with free weights (barbells or dumbbells) for maximum results.

Barbell vs Dumbbell

I recommended at the start you stick with a barbell and it will allow you lift more weight quickly and safely. This helps you stay motivated because you are getting stronger quickly. Once you have gained some strength and build a good frame, make the transition to the dumbbell. Dumbbells are great to isolate, mould, shape and define muscles. For me, Barbell vs Dumbbell, one is not better than the other as both are tools to me. It depends on what the end goal is, based on that I will choose between both tools. If I am looking add size to my frame, I will predominantly work out using barbells however if I am trying to define or get leaner I will also work out using dumbbells.

Impeccable form is a must

You can google, "how to perform the exercise (X) with IMPECCABLE form and technique" I want to emphasise that in weight lifting the movement from A to B (you curling the weight or pressing the Barbell overhead) is what builds muscle.

So if the movement ensures the muscle being worked, it makes logical sense to learn and master the technique or form. The heavier the weight you lift from A to B, the bigger and stronger muscle you will build. But DO NOT forget the FACT, movement from A to B builds the muscle. The list below contains the best compounding exercises for lean muscle gain as well as strength gain.

- Squat
- Deadlift
- Bench Press
- Overhead Press
- Barbell Row
- Pullups
- Dips

Summary

In this chapter we covered the fundamentals of exercising. I would highly recommend that you strive for a balance between the 3 types of activities.

- Cardio
- Stretching
- Weight training

This is the way you will avoid boredom, tedious repetition and achieve your dream body swiftly.

Chapter 9 – Balance Nutrition Base

"Simple can be harder than complex: You have to work hard to get your thinking clean to make it simple. But it's worth it in the end because once you get there, you can move mountains." Steve Jobs

To build a lean body and lose fat as well as having a healthy mind, you need a balanced diet. A balanced diet is one that gives your body the nutrition it needs to function properly. In order to get truly balanced nutrition, you should obtain the majority of your daily calories from fresh fruits and vegetables, whole grains, and lean proteins.

However, with our hectic lifestyles we cannot always know what foods are good for our health, mind and body. So to help you I have made a list of super foods that you need to build muscle & lose fat. In the later chapter, as you will design you are eating plan, I would highly recommend having a balanced diet. A balanced approach gives your body the nutrition it needs to function properly as well as keeping the plan interesting and preventing boredom.

Protein

The biggest problem with diets and eating in general is the hunger pains and irritability when we don't eat. But this is where the filling/satisfying power of protein helps. Lower carb diets tend to be higher in protein and fat, protein is more satisfying and suppresses appetite as protein causes the production of the hormone leptin and PYY which is released from the gut in response to food, PYY then sends signals of fullness and apatite suppression to your brain making you feel full.

- <u>Grass fed meat and chicken</u> - Yes, grass fed meat and chicken is more expensive in comparison to mass marketed grain-fed animals, but rightly so. The problematic grains that we should be avoiding are fed to the animals. Isolation and scientific experiments have determined that the ideal grain fed beef ratio of Omega 6 to Omega 3 is around 20:1 whereas grass-fed beef ratio is 3:1. A greater Omega 6 to Omega 3 ratio can cause problems. Grass fed animals almost invariably tend to be healthier and more natural animals in comparison to mass-market animals due to more freedom and less genetic mutation.
- <u>Wild Salmon</u> - One of the best sources of Omega-3 fatty acids that also gets you 20g of protein per 100g serving. Farm raised salmon is, however, Omega-3 deficient: its corn/grain fed. Go with wild salmon.
- <u>Red Meat</u> – Rich in protein, Vitamin B12, Heme, Iron, Zinc, Creatine, Carnosine and even Omega-3. Eat steaks & hamburgers from top round or sirloin, ensure this is grass fed beef.

- Turkey – If you don't believe saturated fat is good for you, try white turkey. The leanest beef has about 4.5g saturated fat/100g, while white turkey has close to 0g (that why it's so dry). Health tip: Eat turkey with spinach & quinoa.

- Whole Eggs – Eggs are relatively inexpensive, even the free range variants. A single egg contains Vitamins A, B2, B5, B6, B12, D, E, Calcium, Zinc, Folate, and Phosphorus. The major takeaway here is the realisation that eggs are very nutritious. There are concerns over eggs and their effect on blood cholesterol. The reason behind this is that 1 large egg boiled contains around 186 mg of Cholesterol and the recommended Cholesterol daily intake is around 250-300mg, keeping this in mind 2 eggs alone would take us over the daily limit for cholesterol. However, cholesterol intake's raise cholesterol in the blood, once excess cholesterol is consumed the liver slows down its production of cholesterol. Hence eggs are generally safe depending on your genetic predisposition.

- Fish - Fish is loaded with protein, Omega-3 fatty acids and Vitamin D. Majority of people do not get enough Vitamin D, as it is estimated that two-thirds of the US population are deficient in Vitamin D. Fish such as wild: Tuna, Sardines, Mackerel are an excellent choice for consumption.

Carbohydrates

As discussed in previous chapters going fully low carb may not be the best idea and carbs should be used frugally, intake of carbohydrates depends on your current body and what you are trying to achieve.

At a molecular level all carbohydrates are simple sugars linked within a chain, for absorption this needs to be broken down by the body. More complicated carbohydrate is broken down by the body at slower rates, therefore blood sugar is not raised as quickly, which is good because then the fat storage hormone insulin is not released. Sweet potato and chickpeas are excellent examples of 'slow carbs'. Others include:

- Yogurt – Contains bacteria that improves your gastrointestinal health. Get plain low-fat yogurt. Eat it with berries.
- Quinoa – Quinoa is higher in fibre & protein than rice or oats, tastes a lot better and is gluten free.
- Oats – Reduce cholesterol, provide you with low glycaemic index carbs for energy and are high in fibre.

Fruit

Studies have shown all over the world that people who eat more fruits and vegetables as part of an overall healthy diet are likely to have a reduced risk of some chronic diseases. Fruit has been recognized as a good source of vitamins and minerals and for their role in preventing Vitamin C and Vitamin A deficiency. Fruits provide nutrients vital for health and maintenance of your body. The nutrients in fruit are vital for health and maintenance of your body. The potassium in fruit can reduce your risk of heart disease and stroke. Potassium may also reduce the risk of developing kidney stones and help to decrease bone loss as you age.

- Oranges – Contain Vitamin C to fight diseases, magnesium to lower blood pressure, antioxidant beta-carotenes and much more. Quit drinking processed orange juice, eat oranges or make your own orange juice.

- Apples – Apples are also the strongest antioxidant after cranberries. Pectin in apples help weight loss by increasing satiety.

- Berries – Contain strong antioxidants that prevent cancer, heart and eye diseases. Any kind of berries work cranberries, raspberries, blackberries, blueberries, etc.

Vegetables

Nutrient differences cause various problems in almost every area of the body. I.e. Vitamin C helps keep your gums healthy. It is important to obtain all major vitamins and minerals to avoid differences. The answer is to eat Vegetables and lots of them. Although this list is quite seasonal and depends on where you live, a good indicator is a bright colour. Vegetables give you energy and stop tiredness, they also have a lot of fibre to keep you fuller for longer. However, one common problem is limited shelf life as once they reach the supermarket they lose nutrients. You can also use the power of Internet and make sure to stock up at regular interval. All major supermarkets are offering delivery services so the excuse **"I don't have the time or it goes OFF quickly** "is not good enough.

- <u>Carrots</u> – Carrots are also rich in fibre, low calorie and taste good, even raw. Their high vitamin A content improves eye health, especially night vision.
- <u>Tomatoes</u> – The lycopene in tomato paste is 4 times more bioavailable than in fresh tomatoes. Have pizza or pasta with tomato sauce and olive oil post strength training. They are also high in lycopene, which prevents cancer.
- <u>Broccoli</u> – High in cancer-fighting phytochemicals and anti-estrogenic indoles. Broccoli is also high in soluble fibre and low calorie, helping fat loss.
- <u>Spinach</u> – Spinach prevents muscle & bone loss, spinach also prevents cancer and heart diseases because of its high nutrient profile. One of the most alkaline foods.

Fats

- Liquid Oils: Extra-Virgin Olive Oil, Coconut Oil,
- Nuts: Pecans, Almonds, Walnuts, Hazelnuts, Cashews, and Peanuts.
- Cottage Cheese

Nuts

Nuts and seeds are super healthy and most of us, aren't eating enough of them. They are a great natural source of vitamins, minerals, protein, fat and fibre.

- Almonds have as much calcium as milk and contain magnesium, vitamin E, selenium and lots of fibre. They can lower cholesterol and help prevent cancer.

- Walnuts are extremely good for your heart and brain and contain ellagic acid a cancer-fighting antioxidant.

- Pecans have tons of vitamins and minerals like Vitamins E and A, folic acid, calcium, magnesium, copper, phosphorus, potassium, manganese, B vitamins, and zinc. And they help lower cholesterol.

- Brazil Nuts are a good source of protein, copper, niacin, magnesium, fiber, vitamin E, and a great source of selenium.

- Cedar Nuts/Pine Nuts have Vitamins A, B, D, E, P and contain 70% of your body's required amino acids.

- Cashews are rich in minerals like copper, magnesium, zinc, iron and biotin. They are actually a low-fat nut and like olive oil, they have a high concentration of oleic acid, which is good for your heart.

Seeds

- Flax seed is definitely at the top of my list. Two tablespoons of ground flax seed per day is ideal and easy to add to oatmeal or smoothies. Flax seeds are super anti-oxidants that help fight cancer. It also contains a lot of fibre and can reduce your risk of heart disease, stroke, and diabetes.

- Chia Seeds are incredibly healthy seeds rich in omega-3 oils, protein, anti-oxidants, calcium, and fibre.

- Hemp seeds are a certified superfood with cancer and heart disease prevention properties. They are high in protein and fibre with balanced Omega 3 and 6 fatty acids.

- Sunflower seeds also help prevent heart disease and cancer with phytochemicals: Folate, Vitamin E, Selenium, and Copper.

- Pumpkin Seeds are great for your immune system with lots of antioxidants, omega-3 fatty acids, and zinc.

Oils

- <u>Coconut oil</u>- Coconut oil reduces inflammation and arthritis according to a study in India, it can also help fight tumours as it produces ketones within digestion meaning that tumour cells are not able to access the energy. It is also a powerful tool for fat loss as it contains MCFA's i.e. Medium-chain fatty acids in comparison to Long chain fatty acids (LCFSs). MCFAS are anti-fungal, anti-microbial and much easier to digest.

- <u>Olive oil</u> - Olive oil, the extra virgin variety is a great weapon in the fight against fat as numerous studies and trials show more weight loss in comparison to a low-fat diet. As a health food, Olive oil is great. However olive oil could easily turn rancid when exposed to high temperatures which will cause oxidation of unsaturated fats. Overall these oils are very heart healthy, when not exposed to high temperatures.

Drink

- <u>Green Tea</u> – Strong antioxidant and natural diuretic. Green tea also speeds up fat loss, prevents cancer and improves blood sugar & circulation. Drink green tea in the morning instead of coffee.
- <u>Water</u> – Drinking water helps muscle recovery and prevents dehydration from strength training. Get a Brita filter and drink 2 cups of water with each meal.

<u>Summary</u>

This chapter was your health food database. In this chapter we have invested a lot of time and effort researching the best of best foods. I highly encourage you to try a different combination of foods. I would say use the foods mentioned in this chapter like a shopping list or a health database you can keep drawing data (food) from. Use the methods of trial and error to narrow your quest down to a portion of foods which you really enjoy and that are healthy, easy to maintain and provide balanced nutrition to your body.

Chapter 10 –What do you want?

"If you AIM at NOTING
You will HIT NOTHING"

It is vital to have goals in the game of life. Goals give us something to aim for in life, if you do not aim at anything then you will not hit anything. The same principle applies when it comes to exercise and eating healthy. I want you to decide what the end goal is for you. You are reading this book so you are clearly interested in gaining more knowledge. I highly recommended that you set yourself a goal or not even a goal have a vision of what you plan to achieve by being healthy and exercising.

He who says he can and he who says can't. They are both right. Why?

If in your mind, you have a belief that you cannot do something, you physically will not do it. It is as simple as that. Everyone will agree to the statement that,

"We were not born with any of our beliefs".

All of our beliefs were formed based on our experiences during certain situations. For example, as a child, you may have had a dog as a family pet, which was extremely loving and protective of you and as a result, you attached positive feelings towards dogs from this point onwards. Personally I am terrified of dogs. This is because when I was younger my neighbour owned an aggressive dog instead, which one day attacked me. This has caused me to subconsciously link negative feelings towards dogs that most likely will persist throughout your life. Unless I push through my phobia. This process of linking positive or negative feelings towards objects or situations based on our interaction with them begins the moment we are born and continues until the day we die.

- Wealthy people do not hold the same financial beliefs as the poor and middle class.
- Happy people do not have the same emotional beliefs as depressed people.
- Healthy people do not have the same diet and exercise beliefs as sickly or overweight people.

For any diet or workout advice or tip to work for you, you must have a belief that

A) You can drive the plan to completion

B) You must believe it will work

Call to Action

In order to increase your chances of being successful at achieving your goals, a certain protocol should be followed. Please ensure all your goals are 'SMART'. I want you to take 5 minutes to complete this activity, grab pen and paper or open a word document and write down the answer to the questions below.

Goal

- What kind of physical body do you want? Look to model someone whom you admire e.g. I want to be like Hugh Jackman or Beyoncé

Why - Reasons come first, what is your why?

"If you had enough reasons you can do the most incredible things in life."
Anthony Robbins

I encourage you to make a list of reasons to why you want your Goal? It is best to spend some time and write down honestly what you would do if you had your dream body. For the list to be effective, it must be visible to your mind every day to fuel your success. Below are some questions to get you started on your WHY list:

- Why do you want to healthy?
- Why do you want to look like (X)?
- How would it make you feel?
- How would it make your partner or parents feel?

How – How can you achieve you goal, this is where you make a plan of action to follow, in order to achieve your goal.

- How much would you weigh with your ideal Physical Body?
- How many calories do you need to consume to move towards your goal?
- How many meals do you need to consume to move towards your goal?
- Realistically, how can days can you commit to exercising?
- What are the best days during the week for you to commit to your exercise program?
- Do you prefer to exercise indoors, outdoors or combination of both?
- What is the best time for you to exercise: Morning, afternoon or evening?
- How much time can you spend on cardio?
- How much time can you spend on weight training?
- What body parts do you primarily want to improve?
- What is the best exercise for those body parts?
- How many reps per set do you use?
- How many sets per body part do you use?

What – What can you do to ensure you follow the plan to action and don't deviate from your goal?

- What time frame do you plan to achieve your goal?
- Realistically, how can you measure your progress? (Pictures before and after, measurements of body parts)
- How would you know if you are getting stronger?
- How can you track your progress? (A logbook or excel spreadsheet)

Summary

Now you have much better understanding of what you want. I want you to fully believe in yourself that you can achieve it. Why?

Because if you search, you will find countless examples of people with similar circumstances as yours or even worse circumstances and they achieved their goal. So there is no reason why you can't do it.

If you do not believe in your plans, goals, vision and dreams, disappointment will frequently surface. Your lack of belief renders you unable to perceive an opportunity and therefore you avoid taking action.

Chapter 11– Tailored made Eating Plan

No time to plan? A common misconception

"Not enough time for a plan," people say. **"I can't plan. I am too busy getting things done."** A plan now can save time and stress later. A tailored made eating plan will help to ensure you are on track to achieve your goal. There are some qualities in a plan that make it more likely to create results and these are important. However, it is even better to see the plan as part of the whole process of results because even a great plan is wasted if nobody follows it. Planning is an ongoing process, not just a plan. A plan will be hard to implement unless it is:

1. <u>Simple</u> - Is the plan simple? Is it easy to understand and to act on?
2. <u>Specific</u> - Is the plan specific? Are its objectives concrete and measurable? Does it include specific actions and activities, each with specific dates of completion, specific persons responsible and specific budgets?
3. <u>Realistic</u> - Is the plan realistic? Are the goals, expense budgets and milestone dates realistic?

Preparing your tailored eating plan is an organized, logical way to look at all of the important aspects of yourself. Successful implementation starts with a good plan. I want you to take 5 minutes to complete this activity.

Grab a pen and paper or open up a word document and write down the answer to the questions below.

Your grocery budget - If you want to eat better for less think seasonal produce and sales. In order to ensure you gain the results you seek, you must manage your money well. Set aside a budget to fund your eating plan. Each person reading this is unique and has different circumstances so look at your circumstances and then decide your budget.

Do you like choices or do you prefer more structure? Do you want your diet plan to allow room for creativity or do you like the structure of being told what to eat for breakfast, lunch and dinner every day?

Will this plan fit easily into your lifestyle? If you don't have time in your schedule to shop for ingredients and cook complicated dishes, a plan that requires a lot of food preparation will likely frustrate you. You would be better off with a plan, where the food choices are more basic and quick to prepare or you might even try a diet service that offers pre-made, portion-controlled foods and drinks.

Could you stay on this plan for an extended period of time without getting bored or feeling deprived? Make sure there is enough variety and choice. Diet plans that eliminate entire food groups never allow for an occasional treat or require the same few choices each day will usually fail, even for the most motivated and disciplined dieters.

Will your family eat the same foods, or will you (or your partner) need to prepare separate meals for other family members? If you don't live alone, it might be best to choose a plan that the entire family can follow or accept that you might have to prepare separate meals to meet everyone's needs.

Is this a plan, you can follow as long as you like or is there a specific beginning and end point? If there is an end point, do you have a strategy in place that will allow you to ease into a lifelong plan? Ultimately, you want your diet to be a pathway to a sustainable way of eating that will nourish you properly and keep you at your healthy weight for years to come.

How many meals you need to plan for - Take a few moments to think about what you have going on next week. Taking a quick inventory of your plans will quickly give you a rough idea of how many meals you will need to get through the week and how many meals you can get from each batch cooking process.

What you have time for - If you have a crazy busy week coming up, make meals in advance that can be served up in a hurry. I am a big fan of the cook once, eat twice (or thrice) approach.

Create a master recipe list - Having a list of go-to meals is one of the easiest ways to expedite the meal planning process. Consider trying one or two new recipes and use a few old favourites to fill in the gaps. Every time you find a new meal you love, add it to the rotation!

Find a few new dishes to try - Finding delicious, healthy recipes isn't hard, you just need to know where to look. Health-conscious cookbooks and food magazines are great but the internet can literally provide millions of healthy recipes at your fingertips.

Your food mood things - Like the weather, a change in seasons and food cravings can impact what sounds good on any given day. Thinking about these things beforehand will make the recipe selection process faster and meal times easier on everyone.

When you read over your plan and imagine yourself following it, do you feel optimism/excitement or dread? Listen to your gut! If the plan doesn't feel right, it's probably not right for you.

Ensure you record:

- Your starting weight and compare this to your end weight, I recommended checking your weights every 6-8 weeks to see the progress.
- Take body measurements or even pictures to see your progress.
- Record the exercises you perform and track your strength gain.

This eating plan below is an example of a tailored eating plan which one of my good friends is following. He is making significant progress with his health goals:

- Breakfast: Eggs with Oats, orange, green tea.

- Snack: Mixed nuts, pear.

- Lunch: Tuna, roman lettuce, olives, olive oil.

- Snack: Cottage cheese with apple.

- Pre Workout: Black Coffee

- Post workout: Quinoa, spinach, banana.

- Dinner: Chicken, spinach, baby carrots, pear.

- Pre-bed snack: Cottage cheese, berries, ground flax seeds, fish oil.

Nobody has time to cook multiple meals a day, prepare your food for the day while making breakfast or dinner. This takes about 30 – 60 minutes and is key to making this work.

Summary

When It comes to health and exercising, there is no such thing as one size fits all. We as humans are different and have different requirements. So it is pointless following Kim Kardashian's or Hugh Jackman's diet and workout plan because you will not see the same results. I highly encourage you to try out different healthy foods and exercise routines. Through trial and error, you will be able to find what fits or works for you.

Once you have tried a combination of eating and exercise routines and found the one that you like, try to be consistent with routine day in day out. No matter what happens. If you can master consistency in your eating and workout routine, you will see the results. No matter what routine you follow, I wish you great success in achieving your goals. If one routine doesn't get you where you want to go, recalculate and choose another. Consult with your doctor before beginning a new diet plan and reach out to a registered dietician or wellness coach if you feel you need more guidance.

Chapter 12 - Testimonials

This chapter will cover just some of the many people who have transformed their lives. Information about all people is publicly available via multiple sources on the internet. The main takeaway from all of these testimonials is that if they can do it so can you.

Below is the list of people who believed in themselves and successfully changed their health:

- Janet Shore, United Kingdom - Janet Shore was a 58-year-old woman who decided to lose weight after she didn't fit into a normal size aeroplane seat and was embarrassed at the fact she could not fit. Janet weighed 320 lbs at her heaviest and cut her weight down 195 lbs.

"I'm now 13 stone which is about right for me because of my height, my BMI is now spot on and I feel much better." – Janet Shore

- Kirsten Helle, Washington, United States - **"At 25, I was diagnosed with high blood pressure, high cholesterol and prediabetes, but I figured that was the norm because my family has a history of heart disease. Then one day I was sitting on the couch watching my 2-year-old daughter play. I** realized that if I continued down this path, she would follow in my footsteps. Right then and there I decided to create a healthy new family legacy." – Kirsten Helle

- Shanna Fried, Florida, United States - For year Shanna ate fast food and did little to no exercise, which is how her weight had risen to 296 pounds, all this really limited her life experiences. All this changed when Shanna took up boxing which motivated her to lose weight, exercise and create healthy eating habits. Shanna lost 130 pounds, found a career in boxing and now there is no looking back.

"I'm never going to be a 120-pound woman. I'm fit and toned. But most of all, I'm comfortable in my own skin."

Chapter 13 – Final words

DOs

- Record your weight and body measurements on the morning of day 1 of your eating plan:
- Sleep: Try sleeping at least 6-8 hours every day. Another good tip is to create complete silence and darkness if you share a room invest in good quality earplugs and eyeshades.
- Drink at least 8 glasses water throughout the day. This will also help suppress any hunger cravings that may just be thirst cravings.

Life is filled with choices, choices that affect us on an everyday basis, in everything we do, which means our everyday choices are not without significance. Our choices affect us and others in dramatic ways whether we see it immediately or not. There is no such thing as the perfect health code that fits everyone's needs. The perfect health code is what is suitable for you. A tailor made diet and exercise plan is the perfect health code.

Story Time

Sowing and Reaping – There was once a sower, the sower was ambitious and had excellent seed. The sower plants his seed but falls over allowing birds to obtain his seed. However, the sower kept on sowing. The sower knew if he kept sowing, he can sow more than the birds can get. There aren't that many birds.

Unfortunately for the sower, the seeds fell on rocky ground where the soil is shallow. This is not of your making. The seed starts to grow. However, it withers and dies on the first sunny day. However, sower does not lose heart or hope and keeps sowing.

Eventually his seeds fall on the good ground. The sower protects the field and looks after what he planted. Now come harvest time the sower has a large crop.

Moral of the Story – It does not matter what happens just keep on sowing and you will see results upon harvest. Now in order for you to achieve your health goals, you are going to have to acquire persistence in front adversity, failure, family issues or world crisis. In Mother Nature, the farmer plants the seed, looks after it, nurtures it and protects it. When it comes to harvest time Mother Nature gives the famer a beautiful crop for his hard work. The farmer puts in the hard work without any promise of crop on the other end.

You must apply this concept to your eating and workout plan. You will have front load time, effort and energy into it. You may get people whom try to distract you with their excuse. They may even say you are wasting your time; I don't see no results or progress. But just like the farmer who puts in the time with no promise, you must do the same and be persistent when facing any resistance. If you persist and keep on sowing (eating healthy and working out) I promise you will see results upon harvest time. You can't become successful without having many small defeats, frustrations and disappointments.

"It takes up to 4 weeks for you to see your body changing, it takes up to 8 weeks for your family and friends to see, and it takes up to12 weeks for the rest of the world. Keep going!"

I hope this book has been informative and that you can apply these principles and tips to your life. I would love to hear feedback on your weight loss efforts and the book itself.

If you would like to give feedback or comments on the book, please go on my facebook page

www.facebook.com/IPerfection22g

I would like to ask for a favour, if this book has been helpful please share this book with 3 people whom you love and care about and those who you believe will benefit from reading this book.

"May the gains be with you :) "

Hardeep & Raheem

www.ingramcontent.com/pod-product-compliance
Lightning Source LLC
Chambersburg PA
CBHW070123290526
45789CB00005B/2132